GASTRITIS

THINGS YOU SHOULD KNOW

(QUESTIONS AND ANSWERS)

By Rumi Michael Leigh

Introduction

I would like to thank and congratulate you for purchasing this book, " *Gastritis, things you should know (questions and answers)*" series.

This book will help you understand, revise and have a good general knowledge and keywords of gastritis and its effect on the body.

Thanks again for purchasing this book, I hope you enjoy it!

Table of Contents

Introduction..2

Section 1..4

Section 2..6

Section 3..8

Section 4..11

Section 5..13

Section 6..16

Section 7..18

Section 8..21

Section 9..23

Conclusion 24

Section 1

1) What is gastritis?
- Gastritis is the inflammation of the lining of the stomach.
2) What does "itis" mean in gastritis?
- "Itis" means inflammation.
3) What does "gastric" represent?
- Gastric represents the stomach.
4) What is the lining that protects the stomach from stomach acid?
- The lining that protects the stomach from stomach acid is the mucosa.
5) What common bacteria in the mucous lining of the stomach causes gastritis?
- Helicobacter pylori is a common bacterium in the mucous lining of the stomach that causes gastritis.

6) Helicobacter pylori can be transmitted through contaminated water and food.
7) How many types of gastritis is there?
- There are two types of gastritis.
8) What are the two types of gastritis?
- The two types of gastritis are acute gastritis and chronic gastritis.
9) What is acute gastritis?
- Acute gastritis is gastritis that happens suddenly.
10) How long is an acute phase?
- An acute phase is usually less than 6 months.
11) What is chronic gastritis?
- Chronic gastritis is gastritis that happens slowly and takes time.
12) How long is a chronic phase?
- A chronic phase is usually longer than 6 months.

Section 2

1) What cells secrete gastric acid?
- Gastric acid is secreted by parietal cells.
2) What are parietal cells?
- Parietal cells are cells that secrete hydrochloric acid in the stomach.
3) Parietal cells could also be called?
- Parietal cells could also be called oxyntic cells.
4) What is usually the most common cause of gastritis?
- Helicobacter pylori infection is usually the most common cause of gastritis.
5) Can gastritis heal on its own?
- Yes, gastritis can sometimes heal on its own depending on the type and severity.
6) Can acute gastritis lead to chronic gastritis?
- Yes, acute gastritis can lead to chronic gastritis if not treated.

7) Can diseases such as Crohn's disease lead to gastritis?
- Yes, Crohn's disease can lead to gastritis.

8) Can the use of hard drugs cause gastritis?
- Yes, the use of hard drugs can cause gastritis.

9) Can gastritis affect anyone?
- Yes, anyone can get affected by gastritis.

10) Can children also have gastritis?
- Yes, children can also have gastritis.

11) What are the complications of gastritis?
- Gastritis can cause bleeding in the stomach, stomach cancer, etc.

12) What is the function of pepsin?
- Pepsin helps in the digestion of protein.

13) What is gastrin?
- Gastrin is a peptide hormone responsible for the stimulation of the secretion of gastric acid.

Section 3

1) Are signs and symptoms always present in gastritis?
- No, signs and symptoms are not always present in gastritis.
2) What are the common signs and symptoms of gastritis?
- The common signs and symptoms of gastritis include abdominal pain, nausea, vomiting, bloating, indigestion, loss of appetite, black stools, and heartburn.
3) Are the symptoms of gastritis always the same in people?
- No, the symptoms of gastritis are not always the same, they may vary from one person to another.

4) What is the most common symptom of gastritis?
- The most common symptom of gastritis is abdominal pain.
5) What is melaena?
- Melaena is black stool due to the presence of blood in the stool.
6) What is heartburn?
- Heartburn is a burning sensation or pain in the chest.
7) What is pH?
- The pH is the measure of acidity or alkalinity.
8) What is the pH level of the stomach?
- The pH level of the stomach ranges between 1 and 4.
9) What is HCl?
- HCl is hydrochloric acid.
10) What is the function of hydrochloric acid in the stomach?
- The function of hydrochloric acid in the stomach is the breaking down of food.

11) What are some of the risk factors for gastritis?
- Some of the risk factors for gastritis include pain relievers medication, infections caused by bacteria, heavy alcohol consumption, older people, auto-immune conditions, stress, etc.

Section 4

1) How is age a risk factor for gastritis?
- Age is a risk factor for gastritis because the older a person gets; the lining of the stomach becomes thinner.
2) What is erosive gastritis?
- Erosive gastritis is gastritis that causes inflammation and erosion of the lining of the stomach.
3) What is non-erosive gastritis?
- Non-erosive gastritis is gastritis that causes only inflammation of the lining of the stomach.
4) Does acute gastritis always affect all parts of the stomach?
- No, acute gastritis does not always affect all parts of the stomach. It may affect only some parts of the stomach.

5) What is pangastritis?
- Pangastritis is when gastritis affects all parts of the stomach.
6) What are the main regions of the stomach?
- The main regions of the stomach are the fundus, the body, the antrum and the pylorus.
7) What ways can gastritis be diagnosed?
- Gastritis can be diagnosed mainly by blood tests, stool test, and endoscopy.
8) Is there a cure for gastritis?
- Yes, there is a cure for gastritis but it depends on the cause.
9) How is gastritis treated?
- The treatment of gastritis depends on its cause.
10) What are some medications used to treat gastritis?
- Some medications used to treat gastritis include acid blockers, antacids, proton pump inhibitors, and antibiotics.

Section 5

1) What are antibiotics?
- Antibiotics are medications used to treat bacterial infections.
2) How do proton pump inhibitors work?
- Proton pump inhibitors block the secretion of acid by the stomach.
3) What are natural ways to treat or manage gastritis?
- Some natural ways to treat or manage gastritis include eating smaller meals throughout the day. Reducing alcohol intake. Avoiding fried foods, spicy foods, and acidic foods.
4) What is dyspepsia?
- Dyspepsia is indigestion.

5) What is hematochezia?
- Hematochezia is the presence of bright red blood in stool.
6) What is atrophic gastritis?
- Atrophic gastritis is the chronic inflammation of the lining of the stomach.
7) What is hypochlorhydria?
- Hypochlorhydria is a low level of hydrochloric acid in the stomach.
8) What can hypochlorhydria do to the digestive system?
- Hypochlorhydria diminishes digestion, the absorption of proteins and may lead to other health problems.
9) What is achlorhydria?
- Achlorhydria is the absence of the production of hydrochloric acid in the stomach.
10) What is Menetrier disease?
- Menetrier disease is a premalignant disease that causes the growth of massive gastric folds in the lining of the stomach.

11) What is haematemesis?
- Haematemesis is vomiting blood.

Section 6

1) Could tobacco consumption lead to gastritis?
- Yes, tobacco consumption could lead to gastritis.
2) What does smoking do to the stomach lining?
- Smoking can irritate the stomach lining.
3) Can gastritis lead to anemia?
- Yes, gastritis can lead to anemia.
4) What is anemia?
- Anemia is an insufficiency of healthy red blood cells.
5) Can food allergies lead to gastritis?
- Yes, food allergies can lead to gastritis.
6) Can gastritis lead to peritonitis?
- Yes, gastritis can lead to peritonitis.
7) What is peritonitis?
- Peritonitis is the inflammation of the peritoneum.

8) Can bile acid reflux lead to gastritis?
- Yes, bile acid reflux can lead to gastritis.
9) Can ischemia lead to gastritis?
- Yes, ischemia can lead to gastritis.
10) What is ischemia?
- Ischemia is insufficiency of blood flow in a part of the body.

Section 7

1) Can amyloidosis lead to gastritis?
- Yes, amyloidosis can lead to gastritis, although rare.

2) What is amyloidosis?
- Amyloidosis is the abnormal buildup of protein in organs and tissues.

3) Amyloidosis is also called?
- Amyloidosis is also called amyloid disease.

4) What is amyloid?
- Amyloid is an abnormal protein.

5) Where is amyloid usually created in the body?
- Amyloid is usually created in the bone marrow.

6) Can radiation therapy cause gastritis?
- Yes, radiation therapy can cause gastritis.

7) Can traumatic injuries lead to gastritis?
- Yes, traumatic injuries can lead to gastritis.

8) Can burns lead to gastritis?
- Yes, burns can lead to gastritis.

9) Can gastritis cause the malabsorption of vitamin B 12?
- Yes, gastritis can cause the malabsorption of vitamin B 12?

10) What is another name for vitamin B 12?
- Vitamin B 12 is also called cobalamin.

11) Is vitamin B 12 liposoluble or water soluble?
- Vitamin B 12 is water soluble.

12) What are the main functions of vitamin B 12?
- Vitamin B 12 makes the central nervous system work effectively, aids in the formation of DNA, and the formation of healthy red blood cells.

13) What is pernicious anemia?
- Pernicious anemia is when the stomach is incapable of digesting vitamin B 12.

14) What is the intrinsic factor?
- The intrinsic factor is a glycoprotein that allows the absorption of vitamin B 12 by the intestines.

15) The intrinsic factor is also known as?
- The intrinsic factor is also known as gastric intrinsic factor.

16) What is a glycoprotein?
- A glycoprotein is a molecule that consists of carbohydrate and protein.

Section 8

1) What is edema?
- Edema is the abnormal accumulation of fluid in the body's tissues that causes swelling.
2) What are antiemetics?
- Antiemetics are medications used to treat nausea and vomiting.
3) What are antibodies?
- Antibodies are proteins that protect the body. Antibodies fight infection and foreign substances.
4) Antibodies are also known as?
- Antibodies are also known as immunoglobin.
5) What is dysplasia?
- Dysplasia is the presence of abnormal growth of cells in a tissue or an organ.

6) What are histamines?
- Histamines are a part of the immune system that triggers allergic reactions.
7) What are corticosteroids?
- Corticosteroids are medications used to treat inflammation.
8) Can the use of corticosteroids increase the chances of developing gastritis?
- Yes, the use of corticosteroids can increase the chances of developing gastritis.
9) Corticosteroids could also be called?
- Corticosteroids could also be called steroids.

Section 9

1) Does stress-induced gastritis usually cause inflammation of the stomach?
- No, stress-induced gastritis does not usually cause inflammation of the stomach.
2) What causes stress-induced gastritis?
- Stress-induced gastritis can be caused by stress, anxiety, etc.
3) Does eating always improve gastritis pain?
- No, eating does not always improve gastritis pain.
4) Can eating improve gastritis pain?
- Yes, eating can improve gastritis pain.

Conclusion

Thank you again for purchasing this book. I hope it has helped you in your journey to understanding gastritis and how it affects the body.

Please, if you enjoyed this book, I would like you to rate and comment. It'd be appreciated.

Thank you.

www.ingramcontent.com/pod-product-compliance
Lightning Source LLC
Chambersburg PA
CBHW030046230526
45472CB00005B/1704